I0435304

Change Your Mindset, Transform Your Life

By

Dr. Marco Ferrucci

ISBN-10:1497536278
ISBN-13:9781497536272

DEDICATION

This book is dedicated to my mother, sisters, aunts, uncles, cousins and friends. There are too many of you to name individually, but you all know who you are. You have had such an important impact on my life. Your love and support have always kept me focused, motivated and gracious.

Change your Mindset, Transform your Life

CONTENTS

ACKNOWLEDGMENTS

Being the first person to set me on a path towards health and wellness, the late John Stibinger introduced me to exercise and fitness when I was sixteen years old. Since then, I have been blessed with several amazing mentors in my life that have helped guide me to where I am today.

Thank you to Drs. Dean Depice, Nicholas Stabile, Matthew Antonucci, Don and Deed Harrison, Robert Melillo, Ted Carrick and all associate professors at the Carrick Institute and Apex Energetics. Without their guidance and education, I would have never learned the information that is shared in this book.

Another special thanks goes out to Dr. Eric Zielinski for his professionalism and expertise throughout the editing process.

Change your Mindset, Transform your Life

ABOUT THE AUTHOR

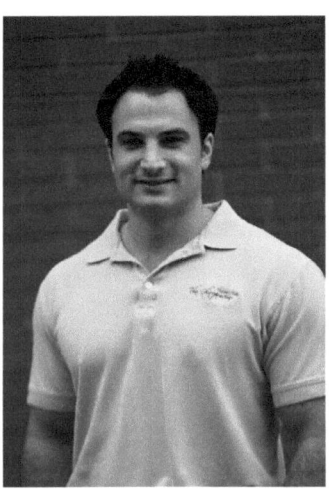

Dr. Marco Ferrucci holds a Doctor of Chiropractor degree. His expertise is in the area health and wellness, with a focus on everything from chiropractic care, functional neurology and fitness to metabolic and childhood developmental disorders. He strives to be his patients' source for optimal health.

Some of his many accomplishments include partnering on two Chiropractic offices, being featured as a chiropractic and posture specialist on NJTV and News12 New Jersey, becoming an adjunct professor at William Paterson University, and hosting a monthly webinar series called "Get to the Source with Dr. Marco. "

You can follow his work by searching "The Chiropractic Source" on Facebook, Twitter, YouTube and Google Plus.

Change your Mindset, Transform your Life

I. INTRODUCTION

My motivation to write this book comes from a frustration that I have with our current health care model. This system is extremely flawed, yet most people do not realize it! Unfortunately, this keeps our society from being the healthiest it can be and countless people are on a path towards sickness and disease instead of **health** and ***wellness***.

Throughout this book, I will be posing questions aimed at having you think differently about health care. In addition, I will educate you on the stressors to health and provide easy, practical tips that can be implemented in your health and wellness plan.

So why do YOU think our society is so unhealthy?

From my experience, I have observed that America's ill health stems from a lack of knowledge about true health care practices. This can even be traced back to improper education in the early years of life.

Here's an interesting fact that highlights my point: Were you aware that Americans spend the most amount of money on their health care and consume upwards of 70% of all the medication in the world? Yet when compared to the other industrialized countries, America ranks almost dead last in almost every health care marker.

How can that be?

Our country has the most sophisticated health care system, the most educated doctors and the most advanced health care technologies in the world. It does not make sense!

How are we one of the unhealthiest nations in the world?

Most doctors have trained us to think that in order to stay healthy we need to supplement our body's natural health mechanisms with synthetic vaccines, medications, antibiotics or even invasive surgeries. While there is a need for these, there is no reason why they should be prescribed at such high quantities. The medical system has educated us, since childhood, to rely on their methods and have convinced us that we cannot be healthy without their help. Unfortunately, this has disempowered Americans from taking responsibility for their health and most people are unfamiliar with basic lifestyle management techniques that keep them healthy.

You see, Americans take a "symptom-based" health care

approach and have not been taught that it is their responsibility to stay healthy: not the job of medicines or vaccines. Simply stated, our society equates health with lack of symptoms: If you don't have symptoms, then you're healthy, if you do have symptoms, then you're not.

This couldn't be any further from the truth!

The truth is that health is not based on symptoms at all. In fact, according to the World Health Organization (WHO), the definition of health is *"having a state of complete physical, mental and social well-being, not merely the absence of disease or infirmity."*

So, why are we so focused on symptoms?

Is there a media influence?

Is it a lack of education from our doctors?

Is there a pharmaceutical influence?

I believe it is a combination of all of these factors, and the purpose of this book is not only to explain why, but to give you some practical tips that will empower you to experience a type of health that you were created for!

In the coming chapters we will take a journey through the major stressors to our health. The major stressors involved in all health-related issues are as follows: physical stress, chemical stress, and emotional stress. In each of these chapters, I will give you a better understanding of how these stressors affect your overall health and provide easy, practical tips for beginning your journey toward being the healthiest you have ever been.

II. CRISIS VS HEALTH CARE

Most people have heard of a health care system, but I am confident most have never heard of a "crisis care system."

Have you ever heard of "crisis care" before?

In case you haven't, let me define it for you: A *crisis care system* is designed to care for people only when there is a symptom or a disease. It does not and cannot help people if they are healthy.

Does this sound familiar?

What do you think?

Does this describe America's model?

The current mindset on health care is based on managing crisis rather than promoting health and wellness. Basing health on symptoms keeps most people unhealthy and will continue to do so until there is a change in the health care model. In other words, if you don't have symptoms and if you don't need medical attention now, the current system is useless. Basically, our health care model cannot help you get healthier or prevent disease from happening in the future.

On the other hand, true "health care" is more effective at helping you become the healthiest you can be because it focuses on having a balance in all areas of your life. As mentioned earlier, the definition of health is having complete PHYSICAL, MENTAL, and SOCIAL Well-Being. This means experiencing optimal wellness in each of these categories. Health care, therefore, requires you to focus on how your body FUNCTIONS rather than how your body FEELS. Focusing on symptom-management will inevitably lead to a future of sickness and disease. You can only prevent sickness and disease by having a health care mentality, rather than a crisis care mentality, because this will make you more proactive toward your health care.

III. HEALTH STRESSORS

Physical, Chemical and Emotional stress are three stressors that can either enhance or diminish health. Take a moment and think about some of these areas in your life.

Do you have optimal health in each one?

Physical

Are you at the weight you want to be?

Do you have an active lifestyle or are you more sedentary in your habits?

Do you care for your spine and nervous system?

Chemical

How is your dietary lifestyle?

Do you eat regularly throughout your day or are you skipping meals?

Do you crave sweets or have a "sweet-tooth?"

Do you smoke, drink or take prescription drugs?

Do you consume a lot of soda or use artificial sugars?

Emotional

Are you confident?

Are you grateful for the things in your life?

Are you depressed or do you have an open mindset about life?

Do you have healthy relationships in your life or are there some destructive relationships in your life?

If any of these questions relate to you, you have imbalance in your life and your overall health will be affected.

Think of these three areas of life as legs of a tripod. When you have all three legs of a tripod working optimally it is very strong and stable. What happens if one of these legs is damaged or no longer works correctly? The tripod will no longer be strong or stable, right? The same thing with regards to the three key areas of your life that I pointed out earlier. If either your physical, chemical, or emotional "leg" becomes imbalanced, you cannot experience optimal health because YOU will be off balance.

As soon as you realize this and focus on improving all

three areas, your life you transform forever.

Discipline and commitment plus action equal SUCCESS! Remember this and your path toward optimal health will be a breeze.

IV. PHYSICAL STRESS

Physical stress is probably the most preventable stressor to health, yet it is the one that can cause the most harm. Some of the most common physical stressors are: chronic obesity, sedentary or inactive lifestyles and (most importantly) spinal and nervous system stress.

As a Doctor of Chiropractic, my primary focus is based on the structure and function of the nervous system as it relates to all other areas of life. Research has shown that when you take the necessary steps to optimize your nervous system, your health will improve dramatically. Likewise, not doing so, can cause havoc on your overall health, which is why I want to begin with a discussion on the importance of proper spine and nervous system function.

So what is the nervous system?

The nervous system comprises of the central nervous system (CNS) and the peripheral nervous system (PNS). This complex system controls and moderates each and every function in your body. It controls your thoughts, heart rate, blood pressure, digestion, hormone levels and much more. When this system is free of stress or interference, you can function optimally.

The nervous system is the only system in your body that is completely encased in bone. The skull protects the brain and the spine protects the spinal cord and spinal nerves. When your spine is in its optimal position your nervous system functions optimally. Unfortunately, the spine is negatively altered because of our lifestyle and this puts undue stress on our nerves. For example, sitting at desks all day, driving in cars for long periods of time and texting on cell phones does considerable damage to our spine and nervous system. To complicate matters, most people have never been taught how to care for their spine and lack the understanding about proper spinal hygiene. This places even more stress on the nervous system, which ultimately changes your overall body function.

These stresses oftentimes may begin at an early age and are the first steps toward sickness and disease. Here's a truth you should not take for granted: **You cannot be healthy without an optimally functioning spine and nervous system!**

So how do you know if you are placing stress on your spine and nervous system?

Being that the nervous system controls and moderates all body functions, we can look at changes in normal body function for some clues.

Changes in Posture. Being that our nervous system controls our postural muscles, changes in posture is one of the most prevalent indicators for decreased function. Decreased function equals decreased health!

Changes in Sensation. This means that you will start to feel changes in the way that your body feels compared to how it normally feels. You may feel achy, deep, or burning pains, throbbing or shooting pains, numbness and tingling sensations or changes in hot and cold sensation. These are signals from the nervous system informing you there is something interfering with proper function and that it should be addressed.

Changes in Movement. This means that your body will move differently than expected. Examples can be seen in balance and coordination disorders, as well as uncontrollable tremors or muscle twitches. People that you would consider "clumsy" are also representations of changes in movement. The more clumsy or uncoordinated the body is, the more imbalance there is in the nervous system.

Changes in Thought. Changes in nervous system function can also cause you to think differently. For example, depression, ADD/ADHD, obsessive-compulsive disorder, bipolar disorders, schizophrenia and autism all have a neurological imbalance associated with them. All of these disorders can be dramatically improved when there is a restoration to the balance of the nervous system.

It is important to recognize that these physical stressors are not only the easiest to prevent, they are oftentimes the most dangerous. By ignoring or disregarding these common signs you will set yourself up for more physical stress, which just makes the situation worse. Remember, restoring balance to your physical health is the first step toward optimal health and wellness.

V. METABOLIC STRESS

Metabolic Stress can be caused by chemicals and toxins that come from your external environment or dietary habits. Being that we may not have control over what is put in your external environment, my focus throughout this chapter will be on the nutritional aspect to metabolic stress.

This is a key point to remember: What you put into your body on a daily basis will either enhance or destroy your health. Whether your choice is between drinking water or diet soda, or choosing between a bag of chips or an organic apple, your final decision will affect your overall health. Obviously, it would be more ideal to choose water over soda and an apple over the chips, but for some people that can be a very difficult decision.

I am here to tell you that it is OK to struggle with these decisions! It all starts with one healthy decision at a time. Every positive action you take will get you moving in the right direction!

Let's talk about how your body works and why nutrition is important...

Most diseases are due to chronic inflammation and oxidative stress. Oxidative stress is due to the presence of what are called free radicals. Free radicals are very unstable cells in your body that are a result of normal cellular destruction. Unfortunately, in order for these free radicals to stabilize themselves, they go "steal" an electron from other more stable cells. This process, over a long period of time, will cause more cellular damage and is thought to be a cause of most chronic diseases like atherosclerosis, diabetes and cancer. In order to stop this process from occurring the body must use antioxidants.

Antioxidants stabilize free radicals to prevent them from destroying other (healthy) cells. They can be found in fresh fruits and vegetables, green tea and a number of healthy foods.

Chronic inflammation occurs when there is an imbalance of the Omega-6 to Omega-3 ratio. Omega-6 is a fatty acid in the body that promotes inflammation in order to help immune function. Omega-3 is a fatty acid in the body that decreases inflammation in order to help immune function. When these two fatty acids are in proper balance, the immune system function properly and inflammation is held within healthy parameters. Unfortunately, because American diets are rich in Omega-6 (due to the widespread use of vegetable oils and processed foods) and low in Omega-3 (due to not eating sufficient nuts, seeds and healthy wild-caught fish) many people struggle with chronic inflammation.

In order to prevent this from occurring, I recommend eating foods that are rich in Omega-3. Some great sources of Omega-3 comes from fresh fish like tuna, salmon, and sardines, as well as nuts like almonds and walnuts. Since many diets lack these foods, I also recommended an Omega-3 supplement. This will help balance the Omega-6 to Omega-3 ratio and decrease the inflammatory process.

Not only will decreasing chronic inflammation and regularly consuming antioxidants help your body function optimally, it will keep you looking and feeling younger!

VI. EMOTIONAL STRESS

Emotional stress is the most overlooked stressor to health. Many people do not realize that their thoughts and actions have an effect on their overall health. Henry Ford once said, *"Whether you say you can or you say you can't, you are right."* So simple, yet so profound, isn't it?

To be successful in your quest toward optimal health is greatly influenced by your emotional state. It is inevitable that you will succeed at whatever you put your energy into, if you believe in yourself and have a positive attitude.

Additionally, in order to become the healthiest you have ever been, you must take responsibility for your own health. The things that you have done up to this point have gotten you to where you are. If you are healthy and are already living a vibrant life, then you should continue along this path and use this book to help "tweak" your strategy a little to reach a higher level of performance. If, on the other hand, you are struggling to reach your health and wellness goals you now have two choices: to continue on the same path and struggle, or accept responsibility for your health, change your mindset and work toward a goal of optimal health.

Power of thoughts...

Did you know that the way that you think about yourself and others have an overall effect on your health?

If you have a more positive outlook on life, then you will create more positive results. If you have a more negative outlook, than you will create more negative results. Simple as that. For example, a positive person may look at a challenge as a chance to grow and prosper, whereas a negative person may look at a challenge as another stress in their life, which can cause more sickness and disease. It is impossible to transform the life of someone who is not willing to work toward his or her goals.

Also, if you complain about your health, yet you are not willing to take responsibility and transform your life, then you will most likely continue on the path of ill health and you will never reach your true potential. My hope is that you will be freed from this harmful mentality. The truth is that YOU are the only person in the way of becoming the healthiest you have ever been and no one or nothing can be blamed. I want you to understand this, accept responsibility, be OK with the fact that you have not been responsible and be free to transform your life forever.

VII. TRANSFORM YOUR LIFE

Now that you have a better understanding of the health stressors and what they do to your overall health, we can take a step toward transformation.

Transforming your health and wellness, as mentioned earlier, requires one very important thing: **Taking full responsibility for your health**. Do not blame your mother, father, children or doctor for your health struggles. Each and every decision you have made, whether good or bad, was made by YOU.

You have the ability to change this and your chance is now!

Regardless of your age, gender, size or shape, you can change your life forever by taking full responsibility of your health. Once this has been done, you can start the process of becoming the healthiest you have ever been.

So where do you start?

The way to begin this journey is completely up to you. Each of us have different areas of our lives that need to be transformed. Some may need to change one area. Others may want to change every area. Either way, in order to do this, you need to change the things that you are currently doing.

The purpose of this chapter is to give you advice in each area of health to help you become a healthier you. *Let this be a disclaimer*: These recommendations are in no way a recipe for optimal health. They are simply lifestyle recommendations that I have used for my patients to help them transform their lives.

Physical Transformation

Transforming your physical health begins by using your health care professionals as coaches and teachers. Your medical doctor is there to help rule out disease processes that need to be addressed immediately. Access chiropractors and other functionally based health professionals for optimal function. Having these doctors evaluate you will give you the OK to begin your path toward optimal health, and provide a baseline to where you began to compare results. Everyone loves to see their progress; it is what keeps most people motivated. Start your transformation with "markers" to track your progress. If you fail to do this you are setting yourself up for failure because you will have no goal in mind. Some common markers that can be used to measure your progress are: resting heart rate, blood pressure, body fat percentage, cholesterol, triglycerides or other metabolic markers as well as total body weight.

Please understand that in order to transform your physical health you must be consistent with your actions and it may be beneficial to have someone in your life that will keep you motivated. Ask a friend, family member, doctor or hire a trainer or health coach to keep you on track. The more people you have on your team the more successful you will be with your health goals.

Healthy Tips. One of the most effective ways to transform your physical health is through regular chiropractic care. You will want to find a chiropractor that is focused on your overall health and well-being, not just your symptoms. Once you find this doctor, stick with them forever! They will be the one health coach that will always push you to become a better, healthier you.

My ideal recommendation for care is to see a Chiropractor for two to three days per week to receive the fastest and most effective results. I have seen many people come to our office only for pain and this method does not enhance their overall health. It just keeps them at the status quo. Like I said earlier, the "status quo" keeps most Americans unhealthy, remember? So a frequency of two to three times per week is ideal for maintaining optimal health. I personally get adjusted, at this frequency, regardless of my symptoms.

If you equate going to a chiropractor with eating well and going to the gym, then it will make more sense as to why we recommend this frequency. If you want to be the healthiest you can be you, you need to have a well-balanced diet and exercise regularly, right?. Going to a Chiropractor to reach and maintain optimal health also requires a certain commitment. Regular chiropractic care will keep your spine and nervous system functioning optimally, allows your body to adapt to stress better and will keep you stronger and thus happier!

Next, find yourself a "training buddy." This person can be a friend or a personal trainer who you workout with. Find someone who will train with you for the simple reason that they will keep you motivated and responsible toward your exercise program. I would recommend doing both cardiovascular and weight training at a frequency of three to five days per week for 20 to 60 minutes per day. This will keep your body strong and ready to take on the stressors of life.

Metabolic Transformation

Transforming your metabolic health begins when you take full responsibility for the dietary choices you have made AND telling yourself, *"I am no longer going to live like this."* Once that responsibility has been taken, you can make the necessary decisions to transform your health.

Transforming your dietary lifestyle takes great commitment but comes with huge rewards. Many of today's most chronic health issues can be dramatically improved just by making adjustments in dietary habits.

Healthy Tips. One of the best ways to begin transforming your metabolic health is through proper hydration.

Did you know that most people walk around chronically dehydrated?

If you are someone who currently drinks sodas, juices and other sugary drinks, please do yourself a favor and STOP NOW! Replace these fluids with pure, filtered water. If you do not handle water well, you can spruce it up with some fruit. Mixing water with freshly squeezed lemons, limes, oranges or even cucumber is a great way to make it more enjoyable. My daily recommendation for water intake is to consume half of your body weight in ounces of water per day.

Next, you need to change your relationship with your breakfast. There are many people who either skip breakfast or eat a breakfast that is high in carbohydrates. The most common breakfast choices consist of bagels, toast, cereals, waffles, pancakes or a combination of all of them. Beginning your day with these foods will set you up for fluctuations in your blood sugar levels and cause more metabolic stress on the body.

A practice I would like you to consider is starting your day with a high-protein breakfast. This will balance your blood sugar level and prevent the dreaded "crash" seen shortly after high carbohydrate meals. Some good choices in the morning that are "protein-based" are a multi-vitamin shake, eggs, turkey sausage or bacon, chicken sausage or slices of fresh natural chicken or turkey. I personally use a nutritional shake in the morning. Beginning your day like this will not only give you more energy, but it will also prevent chronic diseases like diabetes, heart disease and cancer.

In addition to eating a protein-based breakfast, I also recommend snacking between meals. Now when I say snacking, I do not mean chips, candy or chocolate. I recommend snacking on healthy foods like almonds, walnuts, sunflower seeds or even hummus and vegetables.

This will help balance your blood sugar and energy, and will prevent the crash most people deal with throughout their day.

My final recommendation for transforming metabolic health includes supplying your body with natural nutritional supplements. There are many reports that try to negate the importance of nutritional supplements, but I would ask that you trust in the fact that I have seen dramatic changes in the lives of my patients by recommending the following supplements.

Omega-3 Supplement. Omega-3 is a natural anti-inflammatory. It has the same effects as most non-steroidal anti-inflammatory drugs (NSAIDs) that are prescribed by doctors, except there are no harmful side effects. When you buy an Omega-3 supplement it is very important to read the label. When you look at the source of Omega 3, it should primarily consist of two very important fatty acids, EPA and DHA. There is an ideal ratio of EPA to DHA and they vary from children to adults. EPA is a fatty acid that is important for decreasing chronic inflammation and DHA is important for neurological development and function.

Children should use a supplement that has more DHA compared to EPA (2.6 DHA to 1 EPA), whereas adults should use a supplement that has more EPA compared to DHA (2 EPA to 1 DHA). Ideal dosage for EPA and DHA combined should be 900mg for children and up to 3000mg for adults.

Vitamin D Supplement. Vitamin D is extremely important to our body's function and is found to be at low levels in most Americans because we work indoors and lack regular sunlight exposure. Vitamin D deficiency has been linked to several chronic diseases like osteoporosis, cardiovascular disease, cancer and many autoimmune diseases. You can have your Vitamin D levels checked with a routine blood test. The ideal level for this would be between 35 to 80 ng/ml. Should you be deficient, you would benefit from a Vitamin D supplement. Before I recommend a dosage, let me mention that the best source of Vitamin D comes from the sunlight's UV rays. Depending on the region of the world you live in however, there may be times when days filled with sunshine are limited. Wintertime in many areas of the world does not allow you enough time to get an optimal source of Vitamin D from the sun directly, which is why I recommend a Vitamin D supplement. More should be taken during the winter seasons, but a good rule of thumb is to take 1000 IUs for every 30lbs of body weight. For example, if you weigh 120 pounds, you would require about 4000 IUs per day.

Multivitamin Supplement. Multivitamins give you a source of vitamins and minerals that you are missing from your diet. I recommend a food-based or food-state multivitamin. A food-state multivitamin is one that is made from whole food and not made from chemicals or other synthetic ingredients. This source of vitamin is the most easily absorbed in the body, being that it is made from raw food. These types of vitamins can be found in most health food stores. If you live in a remote area, they also can be found easily on the Internet. When purchasing one, make sure that the label clearly states that it is made from whole food, organic, raw ingredients.

Probiotics. A probiotic is the exact opposite of an antibiotic. Antibiotics have been used to kill bacterial infections for many years. Unfortunately, they are very poor at differentiating between "bad" bacteria and "good" bacteria. When you take an antibiotic, you kill both the good and bad bacteria in your body. The issue lies in the fact that your body is equipped with good bacteria in your stomach that helps fight off sickness and disease.

Did you know that more than 80% of your immune system lies in your gut?

When antibiotics destroy the "good" bacteria in your gut, your immune system weakens. Enter Probiotics.

Probiotics replenish the good bacteria in your body, which aid the immune system in fighting disease. Adding this supplement to your life will dramatically change your digestive and immune functions.

At the end of the day, making these lifestyle changes can and WILL change your metabolic health and will bring you one step closer to optimal health and wellness.

Emotional Transformation

Transforming your emotional health starts with your mindset. You cannot transform your life if you are not willing to do so. If you tell yourself you can't do something, guess what? You will not be able to do it!

In order to properly transform your health emotionally, you must recognize the stressors in your life, address them, and then take steps forward to working through them.

Healthy Tips. A great way to transform emotional health is by using stress management techniques. These techniques may include having a more positive attitude toward the things in your life or having gratitude and "thanking the world" for the things that you have. I recommend doing daily affirmations, in which you take a few minutes a day to reflect on the things you are most thankful for. You can choose to say them out loud or write them down, either way, having gratitude helps suppress depressive or negative behaviors.

For example:

- *I am thankful that I have money to pay my bills!*
- *I am blessed to have friends and family that love me!*
- *I am grateful that I am on the path of health and wellness!*
- *I will change!*
- *I choose a BETTER me!*

Make a list of your own and watch what happens when you say them to yourself a few times a day. It is life-transforming!

Exercise is another great stress reliever and huge component for balancing your emotional state. Regular exercise increases the body's endorphins and serotonin levels. This will increase your mood, increase your happiness, decrease depression and is a natural pain reliever.

Physical therapies like massage, acupuncture, yoga and meditation are also great things to incorporate in your health and wellness plan. Each of these will calm your mind, increase your mood and decrease your overall stress level.

I promise you, incorporating some of these practices will transform your life, and will help you become the healthiest you have ever been!

VIII. CONCLUSION

I would like to conclude this book with some motivational insights. The overall theme of transforming your health is understanding that YOU are the only one responsible for being healthy. You can have doctors advise you of this or advise you of that, but YOU ultimately make the final decisions for what is ideal for your health and wellness plan. When you commit to your health and put action steps in all areas of your life, your life will transform forever!

Always keep in mind that health care is a lifestyle, not a moment in time. You need to be taking deliberate actions every day to bring you closer to your goals. Let me leave you with one final statement.

Treat your body as if it were a high performance vehicle. Give it the highest-grade fuel, keep it clean and always make sure it looks and performs at its best!

<u>Summary of Recommendations:</u>

1. **<u>Protein-rich breakfast</u>**. Start the day with eggs, turkey sausage, turkey bacon, chicken sausage or a multi-nutritional shake.

2. **<u>Snack.</u>** Snack between each meal. Eat good snacks such as almonds, walnuts, seeds, rice cakes with almond butter, or hummus and vegetables.

3. **<u>Eat Omega-3 and Anti-oxidant Foods.</u>** Incorporate salmon, tuna, sardines, anchovies, berries and beans regularly into your diet.

4. **<u>Omega 3- Supplement</u>**
   a. Children: DHA:EPA (2.6:1 Ratio)- up to 900mg/day combined
   b. Adults: EPA:DHA (2:1 Ratio) – Up to 3000 mg/day combined

5. **<u>Vitamin D Supplement</u>**
   a. Evaluation: Should be 35-80 ng/ml
   b. Dosage:
      i. Infants - 800 IU/ Day
      ii. Children – 2500 IU/Day
      iii. Adults – 1000 IU / 30 lbs of body weight / Day

6. **Multi-Vitamin Supplement**
   a. "Food-based" or "food-state" meaning it is made from whole food and not chemicals.
      i. Can be a shake or pills
7. **Probiotics**
   a. Read the label, choose one with more strains and active cells
      i. <u>Strains</u> – the amount of different bacteria in the supplement
      ii. <u>Active Cells</u>- the amount of total bacterial cells in the supplement
8. **Exercise**
   a. 20-60 minutes/day, 3-5 times per week
      i. Cardiovascular (Aerobic)
      ii. Weight-Training (Anaerobic)
9. **Drink Water**
   a. Hydration is key to optimal Health
      i. Drink ½ of body weight in ounces of water per Day.
10. **Get Adjusted**
    a. Chiropractic will have the greatest impact on your overall health.
    b. 2-3 times per week in the beginning and minimum of 1 time per week thereafter.